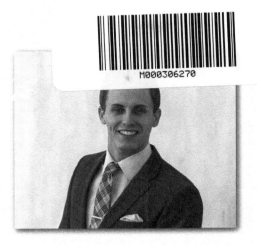

"Doctor, I want to thank you for your professional demeanor during our visit. Your attitude helped my wife with her fear of hospitals and she had nothing but compliments for your conversation and recommendation of her problem."

"Once I met you, I could tell that you were passionate about what you do which put me at ease. Thank you again for the professionalism and excellent bedside manner that you showed during my procedure."

"Dr Matt Koepke took excellent care of my son before, during, and after his surgery. He spent quality of time with us explaining everything. He seemed to honestly care about not only his medical needs but emotional."

ETHICS
UNDER
THE
KNIFE

PATIENT "CARE" AND DISSERVICE
IN THE MEDICAL INDUSTRY

DR. MATT KOEPKE
YOUR VOICE, YOUR SUPPORTER, YOUR SURGEON

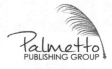

Palmetto Publishing Group, LLC
Charleston, SC

For more information regarding special discounts for bulk purchases, please contact Palmetto Publishing Group at Info@PalmettoPublishingGroup.com.

ISBN-13: 978-1-944313-31-9
ISBN-10: 1-944313-31-1

TABLE OF CONTENTS

INTRODUCTION

What is Culture? Culture is created when a particular group of people share the same values and beliefs. The particular group that I am interested in, and would educate you about, involves the medical community within the hospital setting. The issues created by hospital culture is why this book is being released to the general public. The examples within are encounters I've witnessed during residency training. This book will shed light on the poor patient "care" prevalent today, then become the foundation for an ultimate solution.

In April 2013, an audio recording surfaced on the Internet involving two medical doctors. Their interaction with a sedated patient during a routine procedure was recorded by the patient's phone located in the room. The remarks from the two physicians were outlandish, unbelievable, and difficult to fathom considering their professional standing. The case escalated to national headline news and ultimately, a lawsuit was filed which resulted in the patient winning. This exposure rattled the medical community since the general public had an inside look of the hidden world of the Operating Room (OR)!

To properly set the stage, below is an excerpt from the court record. This is from the Introduction portion of the report, and it reads as follows:

Plaintiff:
D.B. (Vienna, VA)

Defendants:
Anesthesiologist Tiffany Ingham, M.D. (Fairfax, VA)
Gastroenterologist Soloman Shah, M.D. (Fairfax, VA)

"1. This is an astonishing case. On April 18, 2013, during a colonoscopy, Plaintiff was verbally brutalized and defamed by the very doctors to whom he entrusted his life while under anesthesia. Unbeknownst to Defendants Tiffany Ingham, M.D. and Soloman Shah, M.D., their outrageous and appalling conduct was inadvertently recorded. When later confronted with their heinous conduct, some Defendants denied that anything inappropriate had occurred, and implied that Plaintiff must have imagined it since he was sedated and unconscious at times. The Defendants have severely and permanently injured Plaintiff. In addition to compensatory damages, Plaintiff seeks punitive damages so that no other member of the community suffers such egregious conduct when placing his life into doctors' hands."

As a resident physician pursuing a specialty in surgery, the lawsuit had a personal impact greater than I imagined since the majority of my time was spent in the OR. During my training, I had to remain quiet about the examples you'll read throughout the book for the fear of losing my dream career. Unfortunately, this fear of not being able to speak my opinion over-shadowed the moral code I embraced, which stood for patient care. As much as I wanted to vocalize my core beliefs, hospital hierarchy quickly drowned my voice with excuses of seniority: "You're still a resident"; "You're not a surgeon yet"; and my favorite, "This is how hospitals work."

This was not an easy position to be in since my "why" for becoming a surgeon was not congruent with the hospital culture I had always dreamt of joining. Now that I've successfully graduated from residency with the appropriate credentials and have obtained official state board certification license, it is my *duty* to publish this book so we can ultimately strategize together for a solution.

I would not be writing this book if the April 2013 lawsuit had truly woken up the medical community and resolved the issue. Immediately after the lawsuit, I overheard medical professionals voice their opinions by questioning, "How did he get the phone in there?" or by stating, "No patient should ever have a phone on them." This is when I realized we had a *major* issue regarding hospital culture. The hospital culture bred an environment of, "medical personnel are right" and "patients are wrong' from an accountable standpoint regardless of indisputable evidence (i.e., April 2013 lawsuit's audio clip).

As a doctor myself knowing the patient was clearly the victim in the April 2013 lawsuit, it was frightening to be surrounded by professionals who deeply believed their colleagues were not in the wrong. It was also a challenge to trust an environment where the Hippocratic Oath and the morals of hospital culture were not congruent.

Embarrassingly, I was already looking forward to graduation so I could start my own practice and provide patients with an additional level of care aside from just a great surgery. The lawsuit occurred during my second-year of training, which meant, I had two more years until I could pursue this dream.

Everyone can relate to this book because every family has experienced someone who has undergone surgery.

I want to stress that the surgery procedures themselves are not being questioned. I'm solely addressing the culture within hospitals. I believe the issue involves a flaw in human behavior. A flaw in human behavior creates a flaw in the environment encompassed by those individuals which will then become their culture.

I encourage you to read this book in its entirety. It will be difficult because the examples provided will shock you. I purposely began this book with an excerpt from the April 2013 lawsuit to make this as intimate as possible.

My mission is to increase awareness regarding this matter and begin efforts towards the 7.3 billion people (2016 Census) having access to this book in their native language. I am here as your voice, as your supporter, and as your surgeon. We can and will resolve this issue, together.

"Speak the truth and confront the beast or else history will ignore the real issues."

– Anonymous

HIPPOCRATIC OATH

Every medical professional participates in voicing the Hippocratic Oath during his or her orientation. According to Merriam-Webster, "Hippocratic Oath" is defined as "an oath embodying a code of medical ethics usually taken by those about to begin medical practice."[1]

According to Wikipedia, it:

"is an oath historically taken by physicians. It is one of the most widely known of Greek medical texts. In its original form, it requires a new physician to swear, by a number of healing gods, to uphold specific ethical standards. Of historic and traditional value, the oath is considered a rite of passage for practitioners of medicine in many countries, although nowadays various modernized versions are often used. Hippocrates is often called the father of medicine in Western culture."[2]

---

[1] "Definition of Hippocratic Oath." Merriam-Webster.com, 2016, http://www.merriam-webster.com/dictionary/Hippocratic%20 oath.

[2] "Hippocratic Oath," Wikipedia, last modified August 30, 2016, https://en.wikipedia.org/wiki/Hippocratic_Oath.

ORIGINAL IN GREEK

ὄμνυμι Ἀπόλλωνα ἰητρὸν καὶ Ἀσκληπιὸν καὶ Ὑγείαν καὶ Πανάκειαν καὶ θεοὺς πάντας τε καὶπάσας, ἵστορας ποιεύμενος, ἐπιτελέα ποιήσειν κατὰ δύναμιν καὶ κρίσιν ἐμὴν ὅρκον τόνδε καὶσυγγραφὴν τήνδε: ἡγήσεσθαι μὲν τὸν διδάξαντά με τὴν τέχνην ταύτην ἴσα γενέτησιν ἐμοῖς,καὶ βίου κοινώσεσθαι, καὶ χρεῶν χρηΐζοντι μετάδοσιν ποιήσεσθαι, καὶ γένος τὸ ἐξ αὐτοῦἀδελφοῖς ἴσον ἐπικρινεῖν ἄρρεσι, καὶ διδάξειν τὴν τέχνην ταύτην, ἢν χρηΐζωσι μανθάνειν,ἄνευ μισθοῦ καὶ συγγραφῆς, παραγγελίης τε καὶ ἀκροήσιος καὶ τῆς λοίπης ἁπάσης μαθήσιος μετάδοσιν ποιήσεσθαι υἱοῖς τε ἐμοῖς καὶ τοῖς τοῦ ἐμὲ διδάξαντος, καὶ μαθητῇσι συγγεγραμμένοις τε καὶ ὡρκισμένοις νόμῳ ἰητρικῷ, ἄλλῳ δὲ οὐδενί.

διαιτήμασί τε χρήσομαι ἐπ᾽ ὠφελείῃ καμνόντων κατὰ δύναμιν καὶ κρίσιν ἐμήν, ἐπὶ δηλήσει δὲ καὶ ἀδικίῃ εἴρξειν.

οὐδώσω δὲ οὐδὲ φάρμακον οὐδενὶ αἰτηθεὶς θανάσιμον, οὐδὲ ὑφηγήσομαι συμβουλίην τοιήνδε: ὁμοίως δὲ οὐδὲ γυναικὶ πεσσὸν φθόριον δώσω.

ἁγνῶς δὲ καὶ ὁσίως διατηρήσω βίοντὸν ἐμὸν καὶ τέχνην τὴν ἐμήν.

οὐ τεμέω δὲ οὐδὲ μὴν λιθιῶντας, ἐκχωρήσω δὲ ἐργάτησιν ἀνδράσι πρήξιος τῆσδε.

ἐς οἰκίας δὲ ὀκόσας ἂν ἐσίω, ἐσελεύσομαι ἐπ᾽

ὠφελείηκαμνόντων, ἐκτὸς ἐὼν πάσης ἀδικίης ἑκουσίης καὶ φθορίης, τῆς τε ἄλλης καὶ ἀφροδισίωνἔργων ἐπί τε γυναικείων σωμάτων καὶ ἀνδρῴων, ἐλευθέρων τε καὶ δούλων.

ἃ δ᾽ ἂν ἐνθεραπείῃ ἢ ἴδω ἢ ἀκούσω, ἢ καὶ ἄνευ θεραπείης κατὰ βίον ἀνθρώπων, ἃ μὴ χρή ποτεἐκλαλεῖσθαι ἔξω, σιγήσομαι, ἄρρητα ἡγεύμενος εἶναι τὰ τοιαῦτα.

ὅρκον μὲν οὖν μοι τόνδεἐπιτελέα ποιέοντι, καὶ μὴ συγχέοντι, εἴη ἐπαύρασθαι καὶ βίου καὶ τέχνης δοξαζομένῳ παρὰπᾶσιν ἀνθρώποις ἐς τὸν αἰεὶ χρόνον: παραβαίνοντι δὲ καὶ ἐπιορκέοντι, τἀναντία τούτων.[3]

---

[3] Ludwig Edelstein, The Hippocratic Oath: Text, Translation and Interpretation (Baltimore: Johns Hopkins University Press, 1943), 56.

ENGLISH TRANSLATION

I swear by Apollo The Healer, by Asclepius, by Hygieia, by Panacea, and by all the Gods and Goddesses, making them my witnesses, that I will carry out, according to my ability and judgment, this oath and this indenture.

To hold my teacher in this art equal to my own parents; to make him partner in my livelihood; when he is in need of money to share mine with him; to consider his family as my own brothers, and to teach them this art, if they want to learn it, without fee or indenture; to impart precept, oral instruction, and all other instruction to my own sons, the sons of my teacher, and to indentured pupils who have taken the physician's oath, but to nobody else.

I will use treatment to help the sick according to my ability and judgment, but never with a view to injury and wrong-doing. Neither will I administer a poison to anybody when asked to do so, nor will I suggest such a course. Similarly, I will not give to a woman a pessary to cause abortion. But I will keep pure and holy both my life and my art. I will not use the knife, not even, verily, on sufferers from stone, but I will give place to such as are craftsmen therein.

Into whatsoever houses I enter, I will enter to help the sick, and I will abstain from all intentional wrong-doing and harm, especially from abusing the bodies of man or woman, bond or free. And whatsoever I shall see or hear in the course of my profession, as well as outside my profession in my intercourse with men, if it be what should not be published abroad, I will never divulge, holding such things to be holy secrets.

Now if I carry out this oath, and break it not, may I gain for ever reputation among all men for my life and for my art; but if I transgress it and forswear myself, may the opposite befall me.[4]

---

[4] Ludwig Edelstein, The Hippocratic Oath: Text, Translation and Interpretation (Baltimore: Johns Hopkins University Press, 1943), 56.

MODERN VERSION

I swear to fulfill, to the best of my ability and judgment, this covenant:

I will respect the hard-won scientific gains of those physicians in whose steps I walk, and gladly share such knowledge as is mine with those who are to follow.

I will apply, for the benefit of the sick, all measures which are required, avoiding those twin traps of over-treatment and therapeutic nihilism.

I will remember that there is art to medicine as well as science, and that warmth, sympathy, and understanding may outweigh the surgeon's knife or the chemist's drug.

I will not be ashamed to say "I know not," nor will I fail to call in my colleagues when the skills of another are needed for a patient's recovery.

I will respect the privacy of my patients, for their problems are not disclosed to me that the world may know. Most especially must I tread with care in matters of life and death. Above all, I must not play at God.

I will remember that I do not treat a fever chart, a cancerous growth, but a sick human being, whose illness may affect the person's family and economic stability. My responsibility includes these related problems, if I am to care adequately for the sick.

I will prevent disease whenever I can, for prevention is preferable to cure.

I will remember that I remain a member of society, with special obligations to all my fellow human beings, those sound of mind and body as well as the infirm.

If I do not violate this oath, may I enjoy life and art, respected while I live and remembered with affection thereafter. May I always act so as to preserve the finest traditions of my calling and may I long experience the joy of healing those who seek my help.[5]

---

[5] Hippocrates, trans. W. H. S. Jones. Hippocrates, Volume I: Ancient Medicine (Cambridge, MA: Harvard University Press, 1923), 298–299.

"*I will remember that there is art to medicine as well as science, and that warmth, sympathy, and understanding may outweigh the surgeon's knife or the chemist's drug.*"

– Hippocrates

FIRST YEAR
DON'T SPEAK UP

Every first-year resident physician begins his or her journey in late June or early July, depending on location. The majority would have only graduated from medical or dental school a few months previously. On our first day, we are considered "real" doctors. It is difficult to describe the stress a new doctor faces. He or she is "wet behind the ears" yet has the responsibilities of an experienced physician.

For a first-timer, any hospital's environment is completely foreign. Every interaction is new and uncomfortable, and you look toward your colleagues for support, but they're just as puzzled. The new doctors get lost in the hallways along with the patients and their families.

You're trying to find the patient's room the nurse paged you to or the trauma bay in the Emergency Department (ED), where an injured patient waits for consultation.

There is no form of "easing" into a hospital's world.

My specialty is Oral & Maxillofacial Surgery (OMFS). The general public knows OMFS as a subspecialty of dentistry that extracts wisdom teeth, places dental implants, and performs soft/hard tissue grafting. OMFS also deals with facial reconstruction. If a patient sustained an injury to his or her face, an OMFS resident would be paged to the ED to assess the patient for facial fractures and/or lacerations.

A common scenario would involve a patient who was either assaulted or involved in a car accident. Since the majority of these injuries involve the face, I would receive a page from an ED staff member alerting me to assess the patient in the trauma bay. This would involve a thorough physical exam of the oral/facial region and a CT scan of the face to rule out underlying fractures. After assessing the patient and reviewing the scan, I would document my findings in a detailed consultation note with our treatment and/or surgical plan.

The first couple times being paged to the ED, a new doctor will be so focused on locating the patient and detailing every finding on the patient's face that he or she will drown out external stimuli (e.g., unrelated comments from ancillary staff, physicians, nurses, and technicians). After several consultations and finally acclimating to the new environment, most new doctors will find that external stimuli is not as overpowering; thus, they become aware of that stimuli, which often included unrelated comments. This is where the basis of the book originated.

To my amazement, comments from ED staff were often unnecessary and unprofessional. Often as I made my way through the ED to locate a patient, I'd be recognized as the "facial surgery resident on call" and would be approached by a medical professional. He or she would break the ice by saying, "He [the injured patient] must have been wasted," "That guy's face is mangled," "Bet he was on drugs," or "Bet he deserved that." I would ignore the comments and give no response; in disgust, I would continue walking toward the injured patient.

What amazed me was the mindset of the person making such a comment. Why did a staff member think that particular comment would improve the situation? Surprisingly, the majority of comments of that nature came from medical professionals who were *not* directly treating the patient. From a patient-respect standpoint, it's not acceptable for a staff member to voice a negative remark about a patient who was just injured and who is not present to defend himself or herself.

The second problem I recognized during facial

trauma rotation will undoubtedly resonate with many of you. There are three trauma bays (or beds) in an open room within the ED. Each trauma bay has the capacity to house a patient who has sustained a significant trauma. Once the patient is stabilized medically, family is allowed to join their loved one at bedside. Each trauma bay is separated by curtains, not walls! There is a set of computers and phones next to the three trauma bays where medical personnel review scans, complete consultation notes, or speak with fellow personnel to provide patient updates. There were multiple times when I was repairing a laceration in a trauma bay and I'd overhear a physician and/or nurse reviewing the facial scan and saying aloud, "Wow, that guy's face got smashed," or "Bet he deserved that." These types of comments are made *frequently* with little to no awareness that everyone in the trauma bays can hear!

The issue of professionalism doesn't end there. Before spending hours meticulously suturing a patient's face, I would spend a couple minutes creating a calm, peaceful environment for the scared patient. This helps the patient sit through hours of suturing and be more at ease with the situation. A common scenario would involve a technician or nurse walking to the bedside to "peek" at my work. To my astonishment, he or she would make a comment like, "Looks so much better than it did before" or "You should have seen it before it was fixed," with no regard for the injured patient who is just inches away. It immediately destroys the calmness and peace I attempted to create with the patient. I specifically chose words to make the patient as comfortable as possible, and this medical "professional" who is not contributing to the patient's treatment insults the patient, creates a negative environment, and walks off as if he or she did us a favor!

Folks, I believe a form of this happens every day.

The second half of my first year, I was scheduled for anesthesia rotation in the OR setting. This involved shadowing a certified registered nurse anesthetist (CRNA) and/or an anesthesiology resident physician for the first month; then I ran my own cases for the following five months. At all times, every case was supervised by an anesthesiologist.

Anesthesia rotation is where I first recognized the problems with the OR, whereas the ED was where I first recognized problems with the hospital.

Typically, the anesthesia team is the "fly on the wall" during surgical procedures. We take full control at the beginning by administering medication through intravenous (IV) access to allow the patient to drift off to sleep in a safe manner; then, at the end of the procedure, we take full control, making sure the patient awakes safely and comfortably.

This next paragraph may not seem relevant to the broader topic of this book; however, this high-school behavior contributes to the *source* of the problem.

Occasionally, a relief nurse would enter the OR to give the scrub or charge nurse a break. There would be a friendly exchange of information regarding the case prior to each individual accepting their new role. As soon as the relieved person would leave the OR, one or two members of the OR staff would start to gossip about him or her. I couldn't believe this high-school behavior was happening in a hospital environment.

Back to the book . . . One of the main jobs of an anesthesiology specialist is to safely administer medication to the patient so they can be asleep for the surgery. Certain medications are used to accomplish this. The patient's weight, tolerance, and metabolic status will determine the amount of medicine needed to safely accomplish the goal. The majority of the time, a healthy patient will need more than initially dosed due to high metabolism. Nearly *every time* the patient needed more than average, an OR staff member would comment, "Wow, he must party a lot on the weekends," or "That amount of drug would knock one of us out."

Why does it matter how much medication it takes to safely intubate a patient? I believe everyone in the OR should be focused on the patient's safely and refrain from potentially inaccurate comments regarding a patient's social history. These cavalier, harmful comments are made often and contribute to the overall problem of a hospital's culture.

It's important for the general public to know that hospital culture hints that a first-year resident physician's opinion regarding patient advocacy in this setting has little merit. As much as I wanted to speak up and correct every rude, unprofessional comment, I didn't. I remained silent because I was scared of jeopardizing my job. Nervous that I would get yelled at because I was, "only a first-year." I was indirectly influenced to remain silent.

Please keep reading; you'll discover that even speaking up to defend a vulnerable, sedated patient has no traction.

SECOND YEAR
REMAIN HIDDEN

This is a huge accomplishment! A second-year resident physician immediately gains respect throughout the hospital since the label of "first-year" has finally disappeared. It's such an unhealthy environment to instill confidence in a resident physician considering hours or days ago, he or she was treated differently as a first-year resident physician.

Most programs are set up so a second-year resident physician will go "off service." This means he or she will rotate with other specialists for one to two months to learn their specific medical knowledge. For instance, the rotations may include two months of cardiology, one month of neurosurgery, one month on surgical trauma intensive care unit (STICU), two months of ED, etc. These rotations traditionally encompass the entire second-year before a resident physician comes back "on service." Being "on service" means the resident physician is rotating within the specialty *he or she* has chosen.

Because the resident physician is only rotating with a service for one to two months, he or she is utilized as an additional person to help with the work-load. These departments' staff aren't seeking the new physician's medical advice because he or she has limited knowledge about that specific rotation. For instance, because my specialty is OMFS, I didn't have vast medical knowledge about cardiology or neurosurgery before starting the rotation. That's the principle of rotating in those departments: to learn more. Basically, I helped with admission, discharge, and consultation paperwork. The mentality was to do and to not really speak up.

Cliques are common in most hospitals, especially among nurses. Although every floor and every wing of a hospital is different, nurses will naturally form cliques in those areas. Speak to a travel nurse or to a nurse who floats, they will both agree. There is a sense of unacceptance if a nurse who is usually in the west wing of the sixth floor is notified to be in the east wing of the seventh floor due to a lack of available nurses. The nurse will complete his or her job with dignity and respect; however, he or she will have little interaction with the native nurses because he or she isn't "part" of that wing/ floor. This is another example of high-school behavior that should be intolerable in a hospital environment.

This is one of the hardest chapters for me to write. It illustrates the double standard some medical professionals subconsciously embrace to the patients they treat. The next example occurred while I was on STICU rotation. The STICU houses patients who were in critical care after a traumatic incident (e.g., car accident, assault, gunshot wound). This area of the hospital was particularly difficult for patients' families. They would be by the bed of their injured family member, who may be intubated with numerous IV lines attached to monitors, or even on life support. So you can imagine, professionalism from nurses and physicians needed to be impeccable.

Because there was so much to do during the day shift, rarely were medical personnel standing around talking about weekend events and work gossip. However, the night shift was quite different. In the evenings, medical obligations were not as hectic; thus, there was more down time. So guess what happened? The nurses would gather around the center area to catch up on weekend stories and work gossip. Frequently, the group of nurses and technicians would erupt in laughter within ear-shot of a room full of family members watching over their severely injured relative!

It got to the point where I couldn't handle it any-more. Families would look at me, disgusted that there would be *laughter* in such a critical-care environment. I finally walked over to the group of nurses and polite-ly asked, "Hey you all, do you mind keeping it down? The families can hear you laugh. They probably don't want to hear that during this time." I couldn't believe a twenty-eight-year-old physician had to address men and women who had graduated from professional pro-grams to be quiet in this environment around patients' families.

The group didn't say, "Oh, thanks, you're right. That was uncalled for," or "Sorry about that, this isn't the place for this." I received quite the opposite response. My polite request was ignored with a verbal, "No." In addition, the group members' facial expressions solidi-fied their disagreement with me. This is the environment and behavior that patients, their families, and I have to put up with. *This* is why I'm writing this book!

Imagine this scenario: One of the STICU nurses I described as being rude earlier has a family member in the STICU at another hospital. The same scenario plays out. A group of STICU nurses are laughing with-in ear-shot of the room our nurse is visiting. The room he or she is visiting houses their injured relative. Do you think our nurse would go over to the nurses' station to join them in laughter? No! He or she would be pissed and would seek a physician to handle the situation!

Why is there such a disconnect between these two situations when the principle is the same? Double standard!

What I learned during my second-year, especially during that rotation, is to remain hidden. This is not the mentality a resident physician should have in a hospital environment. However, I didn't have much choice when I get bullied by my "colleagues" for speaking on behalf of the patient's best interest. There is a major issue with hospital culture today. Globally, medical professionals need to reflect and become accountable for their high-school behavior.

THIRD YEAR
TESTING MORAL CODE

As a third-year, I spent the majority of the year focusing on my chosen specialty; thus, I started to see oral surgery consultations throughout the hospital. For instance, I would evaluate a patient's dentition for dental clearance prior to an organ transplant or heart valve replacement. Also, if a patient was suspected to have a bacteremia, I would be paged to evaluate and rule out the dentition as a source of infection. I would have several consultations a week evaluating patients' dentition. The majority of the time, the primary team's resident physician would handle the phone conversation professionally. For example, "This is a fifty-four-year-old male who has a history of aortic stenosis. Prior to valve replacement, do you mind evaluating his dentition?" Professional.

Other times, the resident physician would present the patient in a similar manner; however, at the end, he or she would comment, "Man, his teeth are all messed up. They all need to come out." Then a nurse would see me walking towards the patient's room for the consult, and before I walked in, he or she would make another unprofessional remark regarding the patient's dentition, like, "Ew, have you seen his teeth lately? They are all gross. You're removing them all, right?" I hadn't even evaluated the patient, and these potentially inaccurate comments were stated by nurses and medical doctors who have little to no dental education due to the medical curriculum. This behavior continues to breed a negative hospital culture. Hopefully you're starting to grasp the issue(s).

This next example will bother you, and it happens more than you will want to believe.

After the patients were evaluated for dental clearance, some required teeth extraction prior to valve replacement or organ transplant. Due to the compromised patient's medical status, the procedure would typically be performed in the OR setting. The anesthesia administered would be enough to sedate the patient so he or she is comfortable, but not enough for him or her to need intubation. This depth of sedation is similar to what was administered during the procedure that sparked the April 2013 lawsuit.

The oral surgery team had a patient in the OR who needed his teeth removed prior to a life-altering procedure. He was medically compromised enough that the anesthesia team wanted the patient relaxed, not completely asleep. I was performing the procedure and the nurse had just gotten off the phone with the patient's spouse, which normally occurs to provide updates regarding how the surgery is going and how much time is left. I was the most senior resident physician in the OR, and my lower level was assisting me.

The senior nurse hung up the phone, turned to the OR, and said, "Oh my gosh, his wife is so annoying!"

Without hesitation, I turned toward her and said, "Don't say that in the OR! That is disrespectful."

She looked at me in shock and replied, "It doesn't matter, the patient is asleep anyway."

I quickly corrected her, "The patient is *not* asleep, he is sedated."

There are numerous things wrong with this situation. First, the senior nurse had *no* right to publicly state her opinion of the spouse to the OR. Second, she did not understand the depth of anesthesia administered which is worrisome from a medical education standpoint. Third, she proceeded to convince herself that her disrespectful comment was okay by stating, "the patient was asleep."

Unprofessional comments of this nature occur *frequently* within hospitals. Period.

The next part about the situation solidified the publishing of this book.

After the surgery was completed, the patient was safely taken to recovery. I mentioned the senior nurse's comment to a higher staff member of the hospital hierarchy. This was the response: "You shouldn't correct a senior nurse. Hospitals are run by nurses, and all you're going to do is upset people."

Speechless.

Just because someone has "put in their time," they will be viewed as being right. Another negative contributor to hospital culture.

As an Oral & Maxillofacial Surgery resident physician, I perform several types of surgeries in the clinic (e.g., wisdom tooth removal, dental implants, bone grafting). I was removing tori under local anesthesia (i.e., patient is fully alert, not sedated). Tori are excess bone formations on the tongue side of the lower jaw that look like pearls made of bone.

Tori removal is indicated if the condition impedes speech or if a lower denture (i.e., a lower plate) needs to be fabricated for a snug fit. Patients are referred to an OMFS for the surgical removal of these "bone pearls." When performing the surgery, I will reflect the gum tissue away from the pearls of bone until the bone can be viewed. Then I'll place a metal instrument between the bone I am going to remove and the tissue that I reflected. Then I will take a football-shaped bur to contour the bone to the normal anatomy while protecting the tissue with the metal instrument.

Following these actions, the bone was contoured nicely, and the tissue was not damaged on the right side. The left side, however, had a small tear in the tissue from where my bur had hit it, causing minor damage. I immediately stopped the procedure and took a seat next to my patient. I explained to her, in full detail, what had occurred. I comforted her by explaining that it would be easy to repair, with one or two stitches, and that everything would heal nicely.

She smiled and said, "Thank you for being so honest. It's refreshing to hear that from a surgeon."

I proceeded with the surgery and completed it without further complications.

Afterward, I personally visited the patient's husband in the waiting room, and brought him into the surgical suite. I took a seat and explained to him the minor complication during surgery. He smiled and echoed his wife's sentiments: "Thank you, this usually doesn't happen. Keep this behavior up, and you're going to go places in your industry."

I was honest with the patient for multiple reasons. First, she was trusting me to perform the surgery;

therefore, it was my ethical duty to inform her of anything related to the surgery. Secondly, I wouldn't have been able to go home knowing I kept a detail from a patient and try to get rest that night.

What happened next will amaze you.

After I reviewed the postoperative instructions with the patient and her spouse and walked them out of the building, I returned to the surgical suite and was approached by a staff member higher than me on the hospital hierarchy. The member stated, "I overheard what you told the patient. You know that you don't have to tell them all of that. I wouldn't have told her about the damage to the tissue."

I was *speechless.*

I stood there in disbelief and then replied, "I disagree with you completely, and I will tell every patient face-to-face if there's a complication."

My third year as a resident physician tested my moral code. Getting out of residency couldn't come fast enough. I realized there are several fundamental problems within the hospital system that need to change drastically. This was becoming a serious issue.

FOURTH YEAR
VOICING CORE BELIEFS

The fourth and final year. It has finally come! I was labeled as a chief resident during my fourth year, which meant my actions and words *mattered*. Members higher on the hospital hierarchy would look to me to make decisions regarding surgical plans and to lead the younger resident physicians. This year was utilized to polish my surgical skills and develop habits I would carry into the private sector - if that was the route I opted to take.

Early on in the year, a late-night encounter with a chief attending surgeon with a trauma specialty strengthened my beliefs about the unhealthy issues within hospital culture.

It occurred at two-thirty in the morning during one of OMFS's trauma call months. The patient's injury involved other parts of the face, so we needed another surgical specialty to assist. Since I was the chief resident on call, I was present for the surgical operation. The chief surgeon (not a resident physician) from the other specialty was also present while the intubated patient was being prepared for surgery. I don't recall what sparked this next comment; but one of the OR staff members made a remark about the April 2013 lawsuit. To my dismay, the chief surgeon continued with the OR staff member's comment and proceeded to defend the surgeon and anesthesiologist involved in the lawsuit. This was shocking! There is *clear* audio evidence proving both medical professionals were in the wrong. The chief surgeon stated, "Can't believe that patient was allowed to bring in the recorder." The worst part about it was the other OR staff members agreed with him.

I was appalled and finally spoke up. I responded, "I disagree with you completely. The physicians were caught making fun of a defenseless patient and falsifying his medical record. I'm *so* glad he had it recorded – otherwise, they would have gotten away with it."

His response, "Our job is tough, that's how we deal with stressful situations."

I'd had enough at this point and stated, "Pick another field if you can't deal with the stress," then walked off to scrub for surgery.

This is another major contributor to the negative hospital culture. It's something I've heard countless times from nurses, surgeons, and other staff: that the patient was wrong for bringing in the recorder regardless of indisputable evidence. This is a perfect example of "professionals" not recognizing the principle of the story and instead wanting to point fingers so their medical specialty is protected.

Please be seated while reading this final example.

I had just finished a beautiful dental implant surgery and it was approaching noon. It is protocol that after a dental implant is placed, we obtain a Panorex film to make sure the implant is in the correct location. We have paid assistants whose job is to complete this task. I had politely asked the dental staff member to perform this duty while I printed the patient's prescription. The staff member made a facial expression suggestive of, "Why? It's noon and it's my lunch break" in front of the patient!

Without hesitation, the patient commented, "Your face says it all. You really want to go to lunch and not take this film, don't you?"

The staff member replied, "Yes, I want to go to lunch, but I guess I'll go ahead and do this," and then she walked the patient to the x-ray machine as if *she hadn't said anything wrong!*

This lack of accountability is a weekly occurrence.

I've been told by higher staff members of the hospital hierarchy the reason for this "acceptable" behavior is, "That is how residency works."

EPILOGUE

It was difficult for me to write this book and remind myself of the unprofessional events that occurred in such a "professional" setting. This book is written for the general public and the medical personnel who are not aware of these issues.

I also wanted to remind everyone of the national lawsuit (April 2013) that illustrates this issue so vividly. Unfortunately, we've come to a place where we still ignore these same issues.

Now that I have all the official credentials and signatures from graduating residency and being a state board Oral & Maxillofacial Surgeon, it is my ethical duty to continue to speak, write, and lecture on this topic. The patient testimonials at the beginning of this book are evidence that I do actively instill patient-advocacy in my own practice.

I am here as your voice, as your supporter, and as your surgeon.

My mission is for this book to be a mandatory read as part of the curriculum for every medical professional program in the world. I want medical professionals to understand how to act in front of patients, how to maintain professionalism in line with the Hippocratic Oath, and more importantly, how to have the courage to speak up for the defenseless patient without being intimated by hospital hierarchy.

We WILL accomplish this together.

Always be Great,

Dr. Matt Koepke

GLOSSARY

Attending Physician – A physician (MD or DO) who has completed residency and practices medicine in a clinic or hospital who typically supervises medical students, mid-level practitioners, residents, and fellows.

Bacteremia – Presence of bacteria in the blood.

Chief Resident – Senior resident physician in their final year who has been selected organize the activities and training of the other residents.

Computed Tomography (CT) Scan – Makes use of computer-processed combinations of many x-ray images taken from different angles to produce cross-sectional images of specific areas of a scanned object, allowing the user to see inside the object.

Emergency Department (ED) – Medical treatment facility specializing in acute care of patients who present without prior appointment; either by their own means or by that of an ambulance.

Fellow Resident – Physician who finished residency and decides to further his or her education in a one to two year in an academic setting.

Intern – Resident physician in his or her first year of medical training after completion of medical school.

Intravenous (IV) – Taking place within, or administered into, a vein or veins.

Oral & Maxillofacial Surgery (OMFS) – Specialty in treating many diseases, injuries and defects in the head, neck, face, jaws and the hard and soft tissues of the oral cavity and maxillofacial (jaws and face) region. It is an internationally recognized surgical specialty. In some countries around the world, it is recognized as both a specialty of medicine and dentistry.

Operating room – Facility within a hospital where surgical procedures are carried out in a sterile environment.

Panorex – An x-ray image that provides a full view of the upper and lower jaws, teeth, temporomandibular joints (TMJs) and sinuses.

Residency – Stage of graduate medical training after completing medical or dental school.

Resident Physician – One who holds the degree of MD, DO, DMD, or DDS and practices medicine, usually in a hospital or clinic, under the direct or indirect supervision of an attending-physician.

Surgical Trauma Intensive Care Unit (STICU – Wing of a hospital used for caring for patients who have had a traumatic injury or a complex surgical procedure. Patients with a traumatic injury often undergo surgery related to their injury and need our highest level of intensive care.

Tori – Bony growth in the lower jaw along the surface nearest to the tongue.

Trauma Month – The overall goal of this rotation is to introduce resident physicians to principles of patient evaluation and management, with a special focus on trauma and critical care.